BUSTING OUT

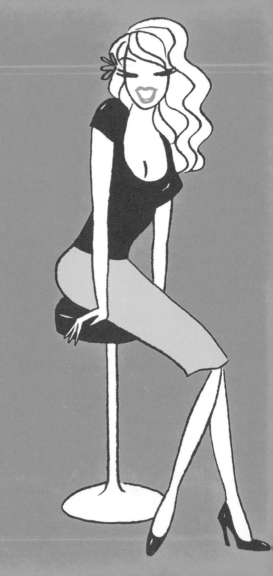

Busting Out

putting your best breasts forward

by **SHIRLEY ARCHER**

illustrations by **NERYL WALKER**

CHRONICLE BOOKS

SAN FRANCISCO

Text copyright © 2007 by Shirley Archer
Illustrations copyright © 2007 by Neryl Walker
All rights reserved. No part of this book may be reproduced in
any form without written permission from the publisher.
Library of Congress Cataloging-in-Publication Data:
Archer, Shirley Sugimura.
    Busting Out : putting your best breasts forward / by Shirley Archer.
        p. cm.
    Includes index.
    ISBN-13: 978-0-8118-5343-9
    ISBN-10: 0-8118-5343-8
    1. Breast—Care and hygiene. 2. Exercise for women. 3. Beauty, Personal.
    4. Brassieres—Health aspects. I. Title.
    RG492.A73 2006
    618.1'90642--dc22

                          2006007594

Decléor is a registered trademark of Laboratoires Decléor, S.A. Junonia is a registered
trademark of Junonia, LTD. Jurlique is a registered trademark of Jurlique International
PTY, LTD. Lucy is a registered trademark of Lucy Activewear, Inc. Pevonia is a registered
trademark of Cosmopro, Inc. Phytomer is a registered trademark of Societé de Courtage
et de Diffusion - Codif International S.A. Thalgo is a registered trademark of Laboratoires
B.L.C. True Cosmetics is a registered trademark of True Cosmetics, LLC. Yon-Ka is a
registered trademark of Multaler & Cie, S.A.

Manufactured in Thailand.

Designed by Sugar

Distributed in Canada by Raincoast Books

9050 Shaughnessy Street
Vancouver, British Columbia V6P 6E5
10 9 8 7 6 5 4 3 2 1

Chronicle Books LLC
680 Second Street
San Francisco, California 94107
www.chroniclebooks.com

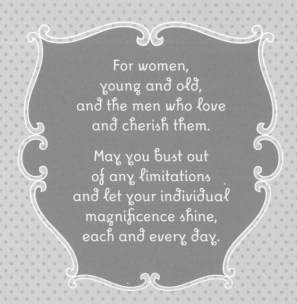

For women,
young and old,
and the men who love
and cherish them.

May you bust out
of any limitations
and let your individual
magnificence shine,
each and every day.

ENORMOUS THANKS TO Sheila Reaves, Jane Iredale, Fabienne Guichon-Lindholm, Maani Fenwick, Joan Timell, Deidre Burke, Katherine Tomasso, Diana Schans, Danielle Wachowski, and Jolene Anello, for generously sharing expert advice on style, skin care, and makeup. Special recognition to Debra Locker for valuable introductions; Maria Argyropoulos for artistic insights; Kay McGuire and Zoran Popovic for photographic expertise; the Ladera group: Lauren Schoenthaler, Noel Hirst, Suzanne Serpas, Susan Swetter, and Dee White; and Morgan LeFahey, Monica Bowditch, and Beth Jolivette for comments. Much gratitude to Neryl Walker for creating perfect illustrations that bring feminine charm, flair, and a little bit of sass. A million thank-yous to Jodi Davis Warshaw for believing in this book as much as I do. Great appreciation to Kate Prouty for keeping me on track. Big hugs to Georgia Archer and Anthony Dominici, my sister and brother-in-law, for their constant support. Much love to René Eichenberger for seeing the unique beauty within me and inspiring me to bust out and share my message.

contents

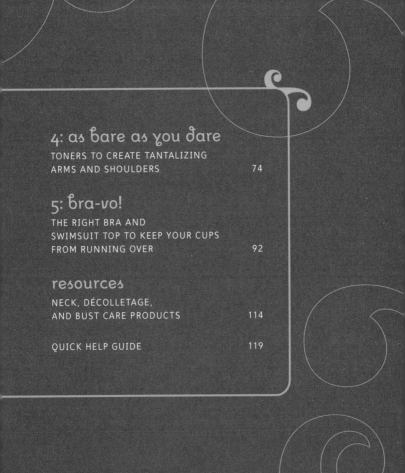

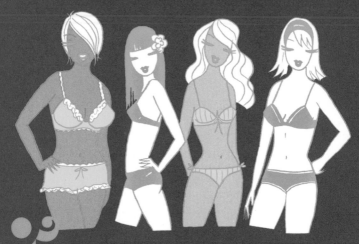

introduction

Breasts are beautiful. Fashion trends come and go, but, like the little black dress, well-kept bosoms—regardless of shape or size—have a timeless allure. From the trim elegance of Audrey Hepburn to the voluptuous sensuality of Marilyn Monroe, it's clear that beauty can fill an A-cup *or* a triple D. The trick is knowing what to do with what you've got and making the most of your unique endowment.

In these pages you'll find a fun *and* effective nonsurgical program to support you in creating your best bustline. I've developed a targeted exercise program for motivated women who want to lift and firm the chest area, and I've gathered tried-and-true fashion advice from top Hollywood stylists. If you follow even a handful of these tips, you—and your admirers—will immediately notice the difference.

It's never too late to address the changes time and gravity have brought to your beloved bosoms. Effective exercises can and do make a difference in bust appearance for all women—whether your breasts are au naturel or have had a little constructive help. During my twenty-year-plus career as a fitness and wellness pro, I've seen women achieve dramatic results by doing the exercises outlined in *Busting Out*. I'm excited that I'm now able to share these secrets with you. Isn't it time for you to take your chest's destiny into your own hands (so to speak)? Let's do it!

In these pages you'll find exercises that perk up breasts, tone shoulders and arms, prevent back pain, improve posture, and help you look sexier and slimmer. Whether you're dealing with postpartum breasts, aging breasts, or breast enlargement or reduction, these exercises will help you look and feel your best. While you're toning and firming, you'll also learn loads of tips from celebrity stylists to help you display your assets in their best light. Today's stars represent more diverse visions of beauty than ever before. Whether their cups runneth over or not, they all make the most of what they've got. And you can too. In these pages you'll learn their treasured tricks of the trade. In addition, an entire chapter is dedicated to bra and swimsuit fit, with fashion-styling recommendations from wardrobe experts that teach you how to flatter your figure and project your personal style.

Breasts are emotionally loaded subjects. Media portrayals of women with skinny bodies and perky, balloonlike, ultra-round, ultra-firm, and ultra-high breasts pressure even the most strong-minded among us to feel that our natural selves are somehow flawed. Those digitized glamazons are simply fantasy and illusion; no woman can achieve such looks naturally. Look at movie starlets throughout the decades, and you'll see beauty in all shapes and sizes. *Busting Out* helps you to feel and be beautiful as *yourself*. Big, small, or in between, your décolletage is a reflection of your unique allure.

Loving and accepting yourself is the first step toward bringing out your best self—a more confident and beautiful you. All the accessories in the world won't make any difference if you don't feel good about yourself. Truly beautiful women glow from within. Many clients ask me, "If I accept myself, does that mean I won't change?" *No, not at all.* The moment when you accept yourself is the moment when you begin to let your individual beauty shine.

Busting Out gives you everything you need to enhance your breasts and celebrate the beautiful, wonderful, sexy, fantastic, fabulous woman that you are. Breasts are, and have always been, *the* symbol of womanhood. Now is the time to reclaim our breasts in all their individual splendor and glory. Now is the time to reclaim all those pet names for breasts and to acknowledge our breasts for what they are—feminine power. Now is the time to bust out of any preconceived notions of beauty and to own the strength of our unique, sexy, and womanly selves. Ladies, get ready to get friendly with the girls and to buoy up your bazoombas!

your breasts
and their many
supporters

What you Got

1

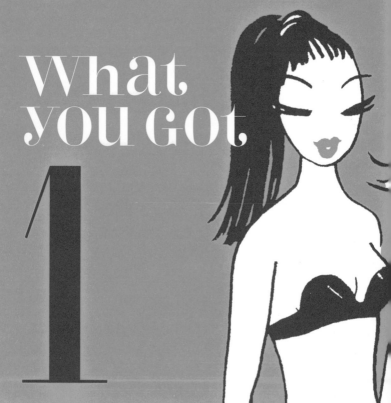

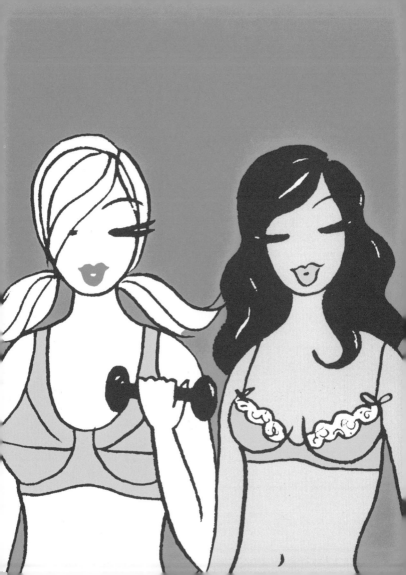

Breasts . . . They've been romanticized, worshipped, memorialized, painted, and sculpted—quite an honor for what are essentially mounds of muscle-free fatty tissue that contain milk glands.

The anatomy of the breast itself is fairly simple. The musculature of the chest wall lies on top of the collarbones and rib cage and beneath the breast tissue itself.

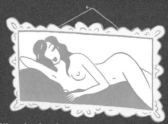

Imagine that the chest wall is like the back of a book rack and the actual breasts are the shelves. Inside each mature breast is a mammary gland, with a network of lobes that produce milk and ducts that transport milk to the nipple. Each breast typically has between five and nine lobes. When a woman is nursing, milk from multiple ducts flows from each lobe and streams from small holes in the nipple's surface like water flowing from the perforated spout of a watering can. The density of tissue in a woman's breasts varies individually and also varies throughout her lifetime.

Breasts themselves do not have muscle tissue, but they do contain fibrous supportive material. These fibrous tissues are known as Cooper's ligaments, named after Dr. Astley Paston Cooper, who first identified them. They provide limited support because they are attached to the tissue surrounding the chest muscles that underlie the breasts. The skin of the breasts also provides a small amount of additional support. Over time, Cooper's ligaments can elongate like overstretched rubber bands, and as they—along with the skin—stretch out, droop results. Gravity and the breast tissue's weight contribute to this sagging, as does excessive bouncing. Therefore, the less bouncing your cha-chas do over the course of your adult lifetime, the perkier they will remain.

To prevent Cooper's droopers, wear a supportive bra appropriate to your size, and *always* wear a structured athletic bra when you exercise. This is especially important if you are pregnant or if your breasts tend to swell with your monthly cycle. Of course, sometimes you *want* to let your bosoms bounce—and on those occasions, by all means do so. For the most part, however, give your girls the reinforcement that they need, and take preventive action to sustain their perkiness. Be sure to check "Bra-vo!" (chapter five) for instructions on how to measure yourself properly, select the right type of bra, and ensure that you choose the right fit. Also follow the skin care recommendations included in the "Secrets of Style" tips to maintain your skin's tone, firmness, and elasticity.

The second-most important proactive measure you can take to preserve or restore the youthful magnificence of your décolletage is to stretch and strengthen the muscles of the chest wall, the back, and the torso. These muscles are the upright supporters of your rack. We all know that as muscles lose tone, they droop and surrender to gravity. In contrast, firm, healthy muscles hold their positions and provide stability.

Surprisingly, a beautiful bustline owes a lot of its aesthetic appeal to strong back muscles and relaxed shoulders. In order to lift the chest, your shoulders should not round forward, but instead must rest in a centered position directly above your hips and below your ears. A wide-open chest and a strong and lengthened waist also provide an optimal backdrop to your breasts. In other words, don't slouch. Avoid rounded shoulders, a collapsed chest, and a rib cage that sinks toward your hips. In the following chapters you'll learn how to strengthen your abdominal and back muscles, which in turn will lengthen your waist.

You'll also learn how to stretch the front of your chest and shoulders to open your chest; to widen your back and stabilize your shoulders; and to strengthen your underlying chest muscles to lift and support your breasts.

To help you put your best chest forward, the *Busting Out* exercise program also includes toners for your arms and shoulders. Reclaiming your arms and shoulders and improving the appearance of your décolletage will lend you the confidence to wear strapless and sleeveless outfits. As you draw more attention upward, be sure to choose the right skin care products to enhance your charms—see page 114 for tips on which ones to use. So there you have it—the right exercises, the right brassieres, and the right skin care are the supporters that will keep you looking and feeling boobalicious. Keep in mind, though, that it's essential to be your own biggest supporter. Once you believe that, you can achieve change; all the other "peaches" will simply fall into place.

stretches to
reveal your rack

loosen up

2

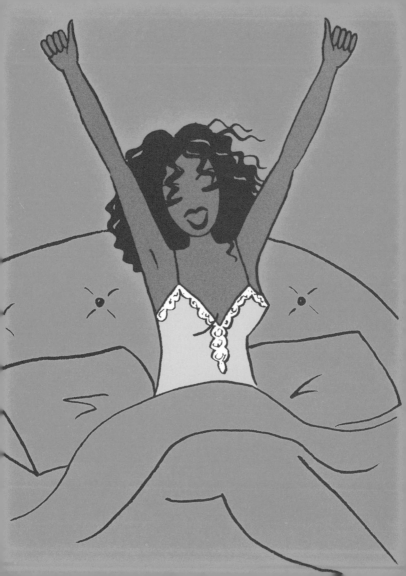

A *flexible body is sexy*. But because today's lifestyle requires us to sit for long periods of time, most people aren't flexible. Instead, they slouch. Their shoulders and chest muscles become rigid and tight, and their back muscles weaken. Daily stretching is essential to correct this muscular imbalance, open up the chest, and restore good posture. Combine stretches with your strength-training program (see chapters 3 and 4) to avoid tight muscles, move gracefully, develop a balanced body, and keep your muscles long. Stretching the torso, in particular, elongates and slenderizes your body and helps to accentuate your curves. As you stretch, remember that an open chest and shoulder area is the hallmark of beautiful bust presentation. You'll enter every room feeling relaxed, confident, and secure.

The stretches in this chapter are easy to fit into any schedule. For example, stretch when you first wake up in the morning, take frequent stretch breaks during the day, and seize the chance to stretch whenever you're waiting in line or sitting at your computer. It's also a good idea to follow each of the toning exercises presented later in this book with a stretch targeting the muscle that you just worked. This helps you to avoid tight or sore muscles and speeds your recovery after workouts.

Breathing and visualization are key parts of good stretching technique. Breathe deeply as you hold each stretch for up to thirty seconds or three breath cycles (a breath cycle consists of one inhalation and one exhalation). Repeat each stretch two to three times, as time permits. With each exhalation, visualize tension draining away from your mind and body. Cultivate an attitude of relaxation and peacefulness. Serenity is always more attractive than stress. A beautiful body is relaxed and fluid; a beautiful face is peaceful.

no. 1

"diamonds are a girl's best friend" overhead stretch

Sit with good posture, shoulders relaxed, and arms at your sides.

* Spread your arms out wide as you reach toward opposite horizon lines, opening your chest. Rotate your palms upward and lift your arms overhead, lengthening your torso. Stretch from shoulders to fingertips as if you want to touch the sky.

* Now gently clasp your hands together. Visualize diamonds on your fingertips. Inhale as you look upward, arch your upper back, channel your inner Marilyn Monroe, and lift your breastbone. To increase the stretch and if it is comfortable to do so, turn your palms forward and up so they face the ceiling. Exhale as you hold the stretch.

* Continue to breathe deeply as you stretch and lengthen your torso for up to thirty seconds.

* For an additional back stretch, lower your clasped hands in front of your chest and spread your shoulder blades wide across your back. If flexibility permits, rotate your palms outward and admire your hands.

* Repeat by spreading your arms wide, then lifting them upward to continue stretching.

secrets of style

FRENCH WOMEN CARE FOR THE DÉCOLLETAGE just as carefully as they care for facial skin. Because the upper chest is angled toward the sun, this area often gets more sun damage than the face, so your neck and décolletage skin can show signs of aging first. To retain youthful skin, take a two-step approach of prevention and repair: invest in a full-spectrum sunscreen with a minimum 15 SPF, and wear an antioxidant-rich cream under your sunscreen to fight the skin-damaging free radicals that are stimulated by sunlight.

titbit

Were Barbie a living woman, she would measure 36-18-22.

no. 2
"come hither" side stretch

Sit with good posture, shoulders relaxed, and arms at your sides.

* Lift your right arm overhead, palm upward, in a long arc until your palm faces downward, toward the left side of your body. Feel the stretch in the right side of your torso. Lift your arm and torso upward and outward to elongate and slenderize your waist.

* Continue stretching through the right side of your torso as you rotate your right wrist as if you're inviting a lover to come hither.

* Continue to breathe deeply as you stretch and gesture for up to thirty seconds.

* Repeat on the other side.

* Variation: To increase the stretch, hold the wrist of your outstretched arm with your other hand. Lift up and away from your hip.

secrets of style

ACCENTUATE YOUR WAIST to magnify your curves. Whether you're short-waisted, long-waisted, or in between, use ribbons, belts, and tailored clothing to create an hourglass shape by drawing the viewer's eyes inward. Highlight the difference between your upper and lower body to create an attractive sense of proportion and shape.

titbit Historically, shaping undergarments were called foundations because of their likeness to the concrete used in building foundations. Women who wore foundations were considered "solid citizens"; women who refused to wear them were known as "loose women."

no. 3

"serene and gorgeous" shoulder rolls

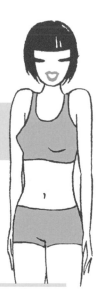

Sit or stand upright with your shoulders relaxed and your arms at your sides.

* Exhale as you lift your shoulders up toward your ears, squeezing the muscles of your shoulders, neck, and upper back as you do so. Inhale and hold the position. Exhale and squeeze your muscles even tighter. Inhale and hold the position.

* Exhale as you lower your shoulders, relaxing your muscles and visualizing tension flowing out of your body like water draining down and away. Relax the muscles around your eyes, nose, jaw, and hairline for a softer expression.

* Roll your shoulders up, back, down, and around, making shoulder circles to further relax and release your muscles. Channel your inner Audrey Hepburn as you consciously lengthen the back of your neck and

lower your shoulders as far down as possible. A long neck is slenderizing and elegant.

✳ Continue for up to thirty seconds. Repeat as needed throughout the day to relax and relieve tension.

secrets of style

INCLUDE NECK AND DÉCOLLETAGE CARE in your daily skin treatment. Neck and décolletage skin tends to be thinner and dryer than your facial skin since it has fewer hairs and oil glands. Use products created specifically for this delicate skin area to refresh, hydrate, and firm. Monthly spa décolletage and neck treatments that include exfoliation and a mask to smooth and tighten skin complete your program, making your skin lovelier and the products you use every day at home more effective.

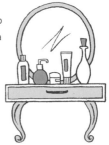

no. 4

"parting is such sweet sorrow" spine twist

Sit with good posture, with your shoulders relaxed, arms at your sides, and feet about hip-width apart, resting on the floor.

* Keep your hips and feet facing forward as you rotate your waist, ribs, and shoulders to the right and bring your left hand across your right thigh. Sit up tall, keeping an open chest as you rotate your neck and look over your right shoulder. Gently squeeze your shoulder blades together to keep your chest open.

* Inhale as you lengthen your spine, keeping your shoulders level. Exhale as you try to increase the rotation, using your left hand against your thigh for leverage. Breathe deeply as

you hold the stretch for up to thirty seconds. Visualize yourself casting long, sexy, lingering glances at a special someone behind you.

✼ Repeat on the other side.

secrets of style

TO BALANCE A LARGE BUST and draw attention to a smaller waist, wear fitted rather than bulky tops. Good fabrics include silk, Lycra blends, soft cottons, and thin lightweight knits. Avoid shiny, clingy, pleated, ruffled, or shirred fabrics, which add volume that you don't need. Avoid overly thick empire waistbands, which can jam up under your breasts and make them look like a tubular mono-boob. Choose tops that lift *and* separate for a shapely body-contouring silhouette.

no. 5
"slinky cat" back stretch

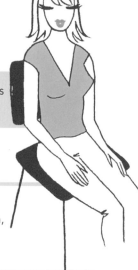

Sit comfortably in a chair. Place your hands on top of your thighs above your knees.

* Inhale and straighten your back from the top of your head to your tailbone.

* Exhale as you look downward and round your back, drawing your navel in, tucking your tailbone, and spreading your shoulder blades.

* Repeat. Breathe deeply and flow through the movement as you round and release your back, cultivating a sultry feline attitude. Continue for up to thirty seconds.

secrets of style

WHEN YOU GO STRAPLESS, choose a stretchy bra that has semimolded cups to maintain lift and separation of your breasts and silicone trim on the top and bottom seams to help it stay up. Alternatively, buy a convertible bra with a strapless feature. Always bring your strapless tops with you when trying on bras to wear underneath.

no. 6

"inner child" back and upper-chest opener stretch

Kneel on all fours in a "table" position, with your hands under your shoulders and your knees under your hips.

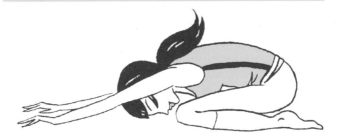

✻ Exhale as you pull in your abdominal muscles and tuck your tailbone under, like a frightened dog.

✻ Lower your hips toward your heels (as far as is comfortable for your knees and back) in the traditional "child's" position. Feel the stretch in your lower back and hips. Walk your fingertips away from your torso, lengthening your arms, with your palms downward. Feel the stretch under your arms, in your upper back and chest, and along the sides of your torso. (Continued)

no. 6 (cont.)

"inner child" back and upper-chest opener stretch

✳ Continue to breathe deeply as you relax your shoulders, neck, throat, and jaw. Keep your shoulders down, and expand your lower back and rib cage as you inhale and exhale. Visualize yourself drawing in fresh energy with each inhalation and letting go of all you no longer need as you exhale. Repeat for three breath cycles.

✳ To finish, lift hips back to the starting position.

secrets of style

WHEN USING YOUR DAILY DÉCOLLETAGE CREAMS or lotions, massage your breasts in an upward circular motion to stimulate circulation, maximize absorption of the products, and give your skin a naturally healthy glow. This is also a perfect opportunity to familiarize yourself with how your breasts feel throughout the month, so you'll know right away if you develop any unfamiliar lumps. Check your breasts in the mirror, too, for any new moles or red patches, which may need to be checked for skin cancer.

no. 7

"queen of the world" chest and front-shoulder stretch

Sit or stand with good posture, shoulders relaxed, and arms at your sides with palms facing inward.

* Clasp your hands together behind your lower back. Keep your abdominal muscles tight to support your lower back.

* Inhale. Exhale as you squeeze your shoulder blades together and gently lift your hands to stretch your upper chest and the fronts of your shoulders.

* Inhale as you hold the stretch. Visualize yourself as Queen of the World, decked out in the crown jewels.

* Exhale as you gently try to increase the stretch by further lifting your clasped hands and opening your chest and shoulders. This counteracts the rounded shoulders and collapsed chest caused by slouching when sitting. (Continued)

no. 7 (cont.)

"queen of the world" chest and front-shoulder stretch

* Breathe deeply as you hold the stretch for at least thirty seconds. Repeat if desired.

secrets of style

LARGE BREASTS ARE HEAVY. Combined with a weak back, they can contribute to an unattractive slouched posture and back pain. If you're very large-breasted and need a strong, supportive bra, try a T-back style or a posture support bra with wide, cushioned straps and back panels. Choose a style with a very wide band and straps so it won't create any back or underarm bulges.

titbit

The word "tits," which first appeared around the 17th century, is derived from "teats" and was not considered a vulgar term until the 19th century.

no. 8

"ladies who lift"
lat and triceps stretch

Sit or stand comfortably. Lift your right elbow toward the sky and slide your right palm behind your neck. Place your left hand on your right elbow.

* Inhale. Exhale as you rotate left at your waist, toward the front of your body.

* Inhale as you lift with your right elbow, drop your chin slightly toward your chest, and lengthen the back of your right arm, the right side of your torso, and your upper back.

* Emphasize the stretch through your waist, and lengthen the space between your hip and your lowest rib. Counter the tendency to collapse into your torso. This stretch provides more space for your internal organs so they can work efficiently. (Continued)

no. 8 (cont.)
"ladies who lift" lat and triceps stretch

✻ Hold as you exhale, and continue to breathe deeply for up to thirty seconds.

✻ Repeat with left arm.

secrets of style

CHOOSE JEWELRY THAT FLATTERS your bustline. Voluptuous women create drama with strong, oversized pieces or multiple necklaces. To draw the focal point upward, wear a pendant that falls at the base of your throat. Fine-boned women look better with a few dainty strands that do not overwhelm their frames. Your face and décolletage are your most visible features when you're seated, and you can attract eyes to your best qualities by choosing the right jewelry and neckline. When you control what people look at, you control what they see.

no. 9

chest-expanding wall stretch

Stand a few inches away from and facing a wall.
Raise your right arm to shoulder height, palm
on the wall. Your right arm can be straight or
slightly bent at the elbow, whichever is most
comfortable for you.

* Step a few inches out with your left foot, and
  turn your torso away from the wall. Stretch the
  front of your chest and shoulder.

* Breathe deeply. Hold for up to thirty
  seconds. Repeat with left arm.

secrets of style

YOU ALREADY KNOW HOW to show off your cleavage. But
for a change of pace and a jaw-droppingly sexy look, show
off your beautifully toned back with a low-cut rear neckline.
Underneath, try a strapless adhesive bra. If you're a C cup
or larger, consider a convertible bra with low straps around
the waist for more secure support.

no. 10
"sexy mermaid" side stretch

Sit on your hips with your knees bent and your legs to your right. Place your right hand on top of your ankles.

* Raise your left arm straight up past your ears. Inhale as you lengthen the left side of your torso by reaching upward and bending slightly toward the right. Lift your ribs away from your hips.

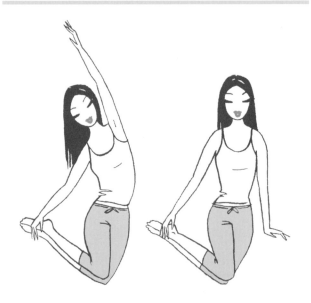

✳ Exhale as you hold the stretch. Breathe deeply and feel yourself growing taller and longer with each exhalation.

✳ Lower your left arm and place it at your left side. Lift your right arm up and over for a counter-stretch as you softly bend your left elbow.

✳ Place your legs on the left side of your hips and repeat on the other side.

secrets of style

TO REMOVE NIPPLE HAIRS, tweeze after you shower, when your skin is wet, your pores are open, and hair strands are looser. If tweezing causes bumps or redness, consider electrolysis or laser hair removal. If you have a lot of nipple hairs that resemble a man's chest-hair pattern, see a doctor—it could indicate a serious hormonal condition.

strengtheners to
lift and support
your love muffins

PERK UP

3

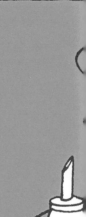

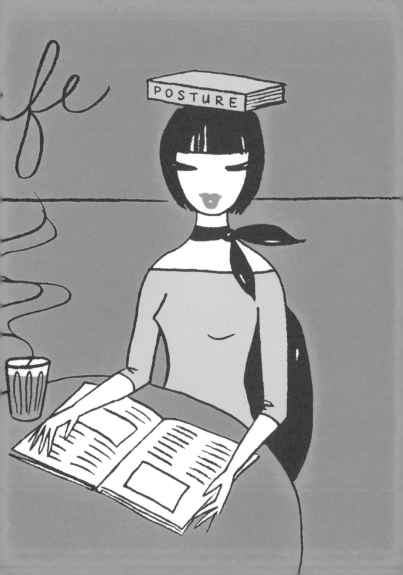

While exercise won't change the size of your breasts, it can, and does, change their appearance. When you strengthen the musculature beneath your breasts—the muscle fibers that lie horizontally across your chest and angle upward and inward—you'll notice a nice lift and firmness. These *Busting Out* strengthening exercises target the muscles that lift your chest, support your back and torso, and stabilize your posture.

Strengthening your back muscles lifts the front of your torso and opens up your chest so people can admire your beautiful bust. You will look and feel more relaxed and confident, which is always sexy. As you do your back exercises, think about the structure of a bookcase. While the eyes may be drawn to the shelves, without a strong backing, the shelves will fall down. The back and core exercises in this chapter build your bust's "backing"—they improve your posture by targeting the muscles that hold you upright.

Posture is key to both beauty and health. Keeping your shoulders down and wide alleviates chronic neck and shoulder tension, elongates the neck, and helps you create ideal posture, which instantly lifts your breasts.

Standing properly makes you appear more confident, slimmer, and taller—some experts estimate as much as five pounds slimmer and an inch taller. Maintaining good posture also tones your deep abdominal muscles—a nice added bonus!

Of course, you have to see it before you can be it. Before you do any toning exercises, see yourself in your mind's eye with perfect posture, using correct exercise techniques and performing every move energetically. Your mind is a powerful training ally. While writing my monthly column on mind/body news for a fitness journal, I've learned that research into the mind's power and the benefits of techniques like visualization and positive thinking is very compelling. You can harness your powers of imagination to improve your bodily awareness, strengthen your mind/body connection, get more effective and faster results from your training, and look and feel your best.

Do these strength-training exercises two to three times a week, unless noted otherwise (posture-check and deep-breathing exercises should be done daily). To increase muscular strength and endurance, perform eight to twelve repetitions of each exercise to fatigue. "To fatigue" means that you cannot complete another repetition with good form—your muscle is completely tired. Start with only one set each. Later, as you become stronger, work up to three sets of each exercise, resting for thirty to ninety seconds between sets. This rest period is a good time to squeeze in a stretch for the muscle that you just worked. Suggestions at the end of each exercise guide you on which stretches work best.

no. 11

posture perfection for instant slimming and bust lifting

Stand with feet hip-width apart. Keep the midline of each foot parallel with the other. Distribute your weight evenly between your feet.

* Straighten your knees without locking your joints.

* Imagine your pelvis is a bucket full of water. Keep your pelvis level so the "water" doesn't spill out the front, back or sides.

* Lift your breastbone upward, lengthening your waist. Draw your lower rib cage inward by tightening your abdominals. Avoid arching your upper back. Do not thrust your chest forward; instead, lift and lengthen, elongating your waist.

* Relax your shoulders. Allow your arms to hang at your sides with palms facing inward. Lengthen the back of your neck, drawing your nose inward. (Continued)

no. 11 (cont.)

posture perfection for instant slimming and bust lifting

✳ From the side, the center of your ankle, knee, hip, shoulder, and ear create a straight line. You look taller and skinnier and your back feels open and relaxed.

secrets of style

GET IN THE HABIT of doing posture checks throughout the day. Invest in a full-length mirror for your home, and check yourself in it frequently until using your abdominal and back muscles to stand and sit in an uplifted fashion becomes second nature. As you become stronger and more flexible, simply standing and sitting with good posture will provide daily toning benefits.

titbit

According to Greek historians, Helen of Troy's breast was the model for the first wine glass. French King Henri II (1519–59) modeled his personal goblet on the shape of his mistress's breast; she was a renowned small-breasted beauty.

no. 12
deep breathing for lift and length

Stand or sit with good posture (see exercise 11) and your arms hanging at your sides. Bend your elbows and place your palms on the upper sides of your rib cage.

* Inhale and exhale naturally, observing any movements in your torso. Do not apply any pressure with your hands. Allow them to rest gently so you can feel each movement.

* With your next exhalation, contract your lower rib cage inward, creating a conelike shape. The widest part of your rib cage is the top of the cone; your lower ribs and waist taper toward the cone's bottom.

* Inhale without effort, keeping your shoulders relaxed as your ribs expand sideways and backward.

* Exhale, drawing the navel toward the spine as your rib cage contracts, which tones your deep abdominal muscles.

* For relaxation, breathe in for 5 seconds and exhale for 5 seconds. You'll look and feel serene and calm. (Continued)

no. 12 (cont.)
deep breathing for lift and length

* Inhale naturally; feel your rib cage expand. Allow air to flow in softly.

---

* Exhale completely and draw your pelvic floor upward as you contract your rib cage. When you lift your pelvic-floor muscles, you will feel a contraction similar to one you feel when trying to stop the flow of urine.

---

* Include at least a few minutes of deep breathing daily to tone abdominal and pelvic floor muscles and to counteract stress.

secrets of style

NO MATTER YOUR BODY TYPE, shape, and size, your clothes look best when they fit well. The label size is irrelevant; cut it out if you don't like it. Find the size that fits comfortably—no binding or pinching! Even if you're rail-thin, skin-tight garments will create bulges and rolls. If a piece doesn't fit perfectly, buy it a size larger and get it altered. A good tailor makes a huge difference. To find a tailor, get references—ask your favorite stores whom they use to hem and alter garments. Take one basic article of clothing for a trial run before you entrust an irreplaceable item to someone new.

no. 13

decline chest push-up for perky pumpkins

Kneel on all fours in front of a bench or sturdy chair. Keep your hands on the ground and place the top of your thighs on the bench or chair seat.

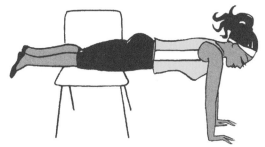

* Slide the top of your thighs across the bench or seat as you walk your hands out as far as you feel comfortable. The farther you walk your hands out, the more difficult the exercise will be.

* Position your hands slightly wider than shoulder-width apart. Tighten your abdominal and buttock muscles to support good posture. Feel your core muscles working. (Continued)

no. 13 (cont.)
decline chest push-up for perky pumpkins

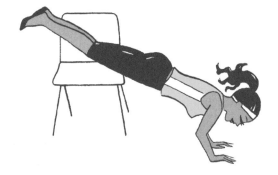

* Inhale as you bend your elbows and lower your chest, maintaining length in your spine. Avoid dropping your head. Keep your legs straight.

* Exhale as you push up through your hands to the starting position. Feel the muscles in your upper chest working; these muscles define cleavage and lift up your chest. Feel the muscles in your back, shoulders, and arms contracting and growing stronger.

* Do eight to twelve repetitions or work up to one minute.

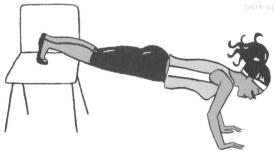

* Variations: To make the exercise easier, allow more of your body to rest on the bench or chair. Or do the exercise on the ground without elevating your lower body. Or place only your feet on the bench or chair.

* After this exercise, stretch your chest and the front of your shoulders with exercise 6, the "Inner Child" Back and Upper-Chest Opener Stretch, and exercise 7, the "Queen of the World" Chest and Front-Shoulder Stretch, to avoid tight muscles that can lead to a collapsed chest and rounded shoulders.

secrets of style

WHEN YOU WASH YOUR BREASTS in the bath or shower, use a gentle moisturizing cleanser. For exfoliation, use a mild scrub, such as sugar, that attracts moisture. If you're challenged by chest acne, use a facial acne-fighting cleanser with a mild salicylic acid or benzoyl peroxide formulation. If your acne doesn't clear up, consult a dermatologist.

no. 14
bosom-boosting incline chest press

Stand in a split stance, with one foot slightly in front of the other and feet hip-width apart. Hold one end of an exercise band or tubing in each hand, with the band behind your upper back. Your palms should face downward. Pull your elbows in toward your waist.

✶ Slide your shoulders down as low as possible and keep them there. Exhale as you press your arms forward and upward at a forty-five-degree angle, palms facing downward. Feel all your chest muscles contracting, particularly in the upper central chest, as you build a strong base of support for your breasts. With each press, imagine pushing any obstacles away as you achieve your toning goals.

✶ Inhale as you return to the starting position.

✶ Do eight to twelve repetitions or work up to one minute.

✳ After this exercise, stretch your chest and the front of your shoulders with exercise 9, the Chest-Expanding Wall Stretch, so your chest muscles will stay flexible and you won't slouch or hunch your shoulders.

secrets of style

YOU WON'T RECOGNIZE YOURSELF with this amazing tip for special occasions: use contour makeup to enhance your cleavage. Shade a half-circle under each breast, and shade up through the cleavage. Darken an inverted triangle between the breasts. Highlight the top of the breasts, the upper chest, and the shoulders with a shimmer powder or bronzer. Light skin looks best with silver or platinum highlighter, medium skin with gold, and dark skin with bronze.

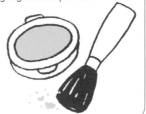

titbit — Numerous mountain peaks are named after women's breasts. The Tetons in Wyoming take their name from French slang for "tits."

no. 15
"focus your high beams" chest fly

Stand in a split stance, with one foot slightly in front of the other and feet hip-width apart. Hold one end of an exercise band or tubing in each hand, with the band behind your back. Your palms should face forward. Stretch your arms out wide at shoulder height.

* Slide shoulders down as low as possible and keep them there. Exhale as you bring your hands toward each other as if you were giving someone a big bear hug. Visualize your cleavage as your chest muscles contract, particularly in the central chest.

* Inhale as you return to the starting position.

* Do eight to twelve repetitions or work up to one minute.

* After this exercise, stretch your chest and the front of your shoulders with exercise 7, the "Queen of the World" Chest and Front-Shoulder Stretch, or exercise 9, the Chest-Expanding Wall Stretch, both of which ward off tight chest muscles.

secrets of style

WHEN YOU PUMP IT UP IN THE GYM, you're pumping up your sexy look when you wear revealing tops on evenings out. During strength training, blood circulation increases and your muscles actually become larger. This pump lends you more muscle definition and size than usual for a few hours. So, just before you head out in a chest-revealing top, do incline chest presses and decline push-ups for lift and chest flies for a defined cleavage.

no. 16
"water nymph" back lat pull-downs

Stand in a split stance with your feet hip-width apart and your left foot slightly in front of the right. Hold one end of an exercise band or tubing in each hand in front of your body. Lift your arms overhead without hunching your shoulders, with your palms facing forward. Pull in your abdominal muscles to support your lower back.

* Keep your left arm elevated as you exhale and bend your right elbow, pulling your right hand down and drawing your right elbow in toward your waist. Feel the muscles under your arm and along the sides of your back contract. Keep your shoulders stable and your chest open.

* Inhale as you raise your right arm back to the starting position.

* Do eight to twelve repetitions or work up to one minute.

* Repeat with other arm, switching your stance so your right foot is forward.

* After this exercise, stretch your upper back and waist with exercise 8, the "Ladies Who Lift" Lat and Triceps Stretch, or exercise 10, the "Sexy Mermaid" Side Stretch. Like swimmers who have strong lat muscles, a toned torso will give your back a slenderizing "V" shape.

secrets of style

SMALL-BUSTED WOMEN, especially those whose hips are larger than their shoulders (classic pear shapes), look great in boatnecks or tops with horizontal stripes at the neckline, which balance out their proportions. Choose tailored, fitted styles. Avoid loose-fitting or boxy shirts that make you look shapeless. Wear big collars, breast pockets, gathered necklines, lace, shirring, ruching, or trimming, and seek out tops with extra fabric and details that add volume to your upper body and create an hourglass image.

no. 17

"watermelon wonders" one-arm back row

Stand in a split stance with your feet hip-width apart and your left foot slightly in front of the right.

* Place one end of an exercise band or tubing under your left foot. Adjust your foot position depending on how much tension you want on the band. Hold the other end in your right hand, palm facing downward, with your thumb on the inside.

* Place your left hand on your left thigh for support. Relax your shoulders and keep your upper body still. Pull in your abdominal muscles to support your lower back.

* Exhale as you bend your right elbow, pulling your hand toward your hip and rotating your forearm so your palm faces upward, with your thumb on the outside. Use your back muscles rather than your arms.

* Inhale as you lower your hand to the starting position. Keep your shoulders stable, wrist flat, and spine in a lengthened position. Challenge your core muscles to keep your torso still as your arm moves.

* Do eight to twelve repetitions or work up to one minute.

* Repeat on the other side.

* After this exercise, stretch your torso and back with exercise 1, the "Diamonds Are a Girl's Best Friend" Overhead Stretch, or exercise 2, the "Come Hither" Side Stretch.

secrets of style

BEFORE YOU GO OUT in a low-cut top, do a quick cleavage check. Stand in front of a mirror, bend over, and check out what you can see. If you're not comfortable with the big reveal, layer a tank or camisole under your top. Alternatively, use double-stick toupee or lingerie tape to secure your top to your chest.

no. 18

"we must firm up our bust" back shoulder blade squeeze

Stand or sit comfortably in a chair, shoulders relaxed and arms at your sides. Hold the end of an exercise band in each hand in front of your body. Tighten your abdominals to support your back. Maintain good posture (see exercise 11).

✳ Exhale as you squeeze your shoulder blades together. Feel the muscles in your mid-upper back working. Notice how your chest lifts and opens wide. Keep your shoulders relaxed, torso stable, and wrists flat. Avoid arching your lower back or hunching your shoulders.

✳ Inhale as you return your arms to the starting position.

✳ Do eight to twelve repetitions or work up to one minute.

* After this exercise, stretch your torso and back with exercise 1, the "Diamonds Are a Girl's Best Friend" Overhead Stretch, or exercise 8, the "Ladies Who Lift" Lat and Triceps Stretch.

secrets of style

SHINY FABRICS ARE VERY FESTIVE for evening or holiday wear. But be careful with the color you choose, since shine attracts light and exaggerates the power of a color to make you look larger. Big, bodacious women look better in deep, dark shiny tops, while small-busted women can balance out their proportions with bright or light colors.

no. 19

"perky peaches" chest and back pullover

This is an advanced exercise, as you use your core
muscles to support your torso and neck. If you experience
any discomfort, wait until you are stronger.

* Lie on your back across a bench or chair with your
  knees bent and your feet on the ground, preserving
  the natural curve of your lower back. Tighten your
  buttocks to support your lower back. Keep your thighs
  parallel to the ground.

---

* With both hands, hold one dumbbell directly over
  your chest.

---

* Inhale as you lower the weight in an arc past your
  head, keeping your rib cage in contact with the bench

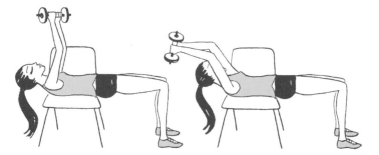

or chair by pulling in your abdominals. Go only as far as your shoulder flexibility permits. Avoid any position that causes pain or discomfort. Enjoy the stretch in your chest and rib cage.

* Exhale as you lift the weight overhead in an arc until your hands are above your torso. Feel your back muscles working underneath your arms and along the sides of your torso. To emphasize chest muscles, bend your elbows. To emphasize back muscles, keep your arms as straight as possible.

* Do eight to twelve repetitions or work up to one minute.

* After this exercise, stretch your chest and back with exercise 1, the "Diamonds Are a Girl's Best Friend" Overhead Stretch, and exercise 7, the "Queen of the World" Chest and Front-Shoulder Stretch.

secrets of style

TO GET A BUTTON-UP SHIRT TO FIT PROPERLY, add bust darts to trim out baggy excess fabric, particularly if you are large-chested. If your shirtfront gaps between buttons, sew a hook and eye or a snap into the placket for a custom fit.

no. 20
"I can fly" back extension

Lie face down with your forehead on the back of your hands, your palms down, and your elbows out wide so your arms form a diamond shape. Relax your shoulders. Pull in your abdominals and tighten your buttocks to support the lower back.

* Exhale as you lift your upper body and arms off the floor, keeping your pelvis, legs, and feet on the ground. Lengthen your spine and lift your breastbone upward, keeping your shoulders down and away from your ears.

* Inhale as you lower to the starting position.

* Do eight to twelve repetitions or work up to one minute.

* Variations: To make the exercise easier or if you're prone to hunching your shoulders, keep your arms at your sides. Lift your upper body as described, keeping your shoulders down and wide.

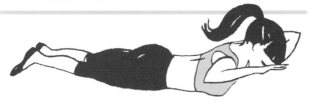

* To make the exercise harder, extend your arms so your body forms a Y shape, with your palms facing inward. Lift your upper body as described.

* After this exercise, stretch your back with exercise 5, the "Slinky Cat" Back Stretch.

secrets of style

SKIN CARE RESEARCH SHOWS that many essential oils contain antioxidants that can soothe, soften, regenerate, and revitalize skin. Antioxidants, found in algae, grape seed, blackberry, pomegranate, and blueberry extracts, combat free radicals that damage skin cells.

Other compounds also promote polished skin and perky ta-tas. To lift and firm the bust, use products with ingredients that contain elastin, such as kigelia africana. To prevent stretch marks during pregnancy, use products with ingredients that soothe and soften skin and promote elasticity, such as chamomile, aloe vera, onion juice extract, and vitamin C. To heal existing stretch marks, use exfoliating products that remove dead skin, as well as skin-regenerating products with ingredients such as idebenone, copper peptides, niacin, vitamin C, and zinc.

no. 21

shimmy-ready
shoulder blade push-up

This exercise tones your core muscles and back and firms up your posture.

✳ Kneel on all fours in a table position, with hands under shoulders and knees under hips. Pull in your abdominals, slide your shoulder blades down toward your waist, and keep your torso parallel to the ground. Avoid tucking your tailbone or arching your back.

✳ Exhale as you squeeze your shoulder blades together without hunching your shoulders. Keep your arms straight without locking your elbows.

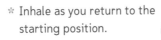

✳ Inhale as you return to the starting position.

✳ Exhale as you spread your shoulder blades wide and

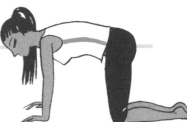

round your upper back without hunching your shoulders. Continue to keep your arms straight without locking your elbows.

* Inhale as you return to the starting position.

* By alternately squeezing your shoulder blades together and rounding your back, you tone up important muscles in your mid-upper back and you learn where the shoulders should rest. This is an important first step away from rounded shoulders and a slouched posture and toward a beautiful open chest, long neck, and relaxed, centered shoulders.

* Do eight to twelve repetitions or work up to one minute.

* After this exercise, stretch and relax your shoulders and upper back with exercise 3, "Serene and Gorgeous" Shoulder Rolls, and exercise 6, the "Inner Child" Back and Upper-Chest Opener Stretch.

* Once you've mastered this exercise, you can use it as a warm-up before your regular push-ups to ensure that your shoulders are in the correct centered position.

secrets of style

USE A MIRROR TO CHECK whether your shoulders are level with each other. Many women develop a one-sided slouch because they always carry their heavy shoulder bags on the same arm. If you need to carry a shoulder bag or tote, switch it between your left and right side to create a more balanced body. Keep your bags light and in scale with your body. Bigger and taller women look fashionable with large bags, but petite people can look overwhelmed. Check out how the bag rests against your body and affects your profile, too: any bag adds width and attracts viewers' attention.

As early as 360 AD, French women sought means to support their breasts with bands of cloth wrapped around their chests. This garment was called a bandeau.

no. 22

"here I am" shoulder external rotator

Stand with feet hip-width apart. Hold an exercise band
or tubing in front of your body, one end in each hand,
with your palms facing inward, your upper arms next to
your torso, and your elbows bent at ninety degrees.
Relax your shoulders and keep your forearms parallel
to the ground. Pull in your abdominals to
support your lower back.

* Exhale as you rotate your arms
  horizontally to the sides until your
  palms face forward, as you stretch
  the band. Keep your upper
  arms locked next to your torso,
  your elbows at your waist, and
  the wrist joints flat. Feel the muscles
  around your shoulder joints working.
  Notice how this movement opens up
  your chest.

* Inhale as you return to the
  starting position. (Continued)

no. 22 (cont.)

"here I am" shoulder external rotator

✳ Do eight to twelve repetitions or work up to one minute.

✳ After this exercise, stretch and relax your shoulders and upper back with exercise 3, "Serene and Gorgeous" Shoulder Rolls.

secrets of style

IT'S NOT ALL ABOUT THE BREASTS! The lines of a woman's neck and collarbones are also very sexy. For added drama, draw attention to your collarbones by applying a cream highlighter with your fingers on top of the bones. Use contour makeup behind the collarbones to make them pop even more. Alternatively, try an aerosol spray-on shimmer for even coverage over your décolletage. And go jewelry-free to show off the simple beauty of your neck. Throat baring is a primitive courtship gesture that means you are approachable. According to social anthropologists, when a woman shows her throat to a man, she is signaling that she is vulnerable.

no. 23

"I am woman, hear me roar" plank

Lie face down with your legs straight. Rest your forearms on the ground with your palms facing inward, and bend your arms so that your shoulders are directly above your elbows. You can clasp your hands to form a tripod if that's more comfortable for you.

* Stabilize your shoulders by sliding your shoulder blades down your back and keeping them low. Lengthen the back of your neck, aligning your ears with your shoulders.

* Pull in your abdominals and slightly tighten your buttocks to support your lower back. Draw the lower end of your rib cage in toward your spine. Avoid arching your back, hunching your shoulders, or dropping your head. (Continued)

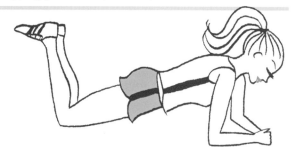

no. 23 (CONT.)

"I am woman, hear me roar" plank

* Exhale as you push up onto your knees. Feel your abdominal and back muscles, as well as your buttocks, working to support your body.

* Breathe normally as you work up to a thirty-second hold.

* After this exercise, stretch and relax your back with exercise 5, the "Slinky Cat" Back Stretch, and exercise 6, the "Inner Child" Back and Upper-Chest Opener Stretch.

* Variation: For a harder version, curl your toes under. Exhale as you push up onto the balls of your feet. Lengthen your body from the top of your head to the soles of your feet. Breathe normally as you work up to a thirty-second hold.

secrets of style

BIG, BEAUTIFUL WOMEN LOOK GREAT in narrow V-necks
and necklines with slits that yield just a glimpse of sexy
cleavage. Avoid puffed sleeves, chest pockets, and any other
excess fabric around the chest. Stay away from big collars,
too. Instead choose single-breasted blazers, small notch
collars, or collarless styles.

titbit

Are boobs simply buns in front? Some
theorists believe that when humans became
an upright species, enlarged breasts evolved
in women as a sexual signal to males. The
idea is that men previously had associated arousal with
the sight of female buttocks. Once we stood up, men
needed a frontal spotlight as well. This may resolve the
long-debated question of why human females are the
only mammals with permanently enlarged breasts.

toners to create
tantalizing arms
and shoulders

as bare as
you Dare

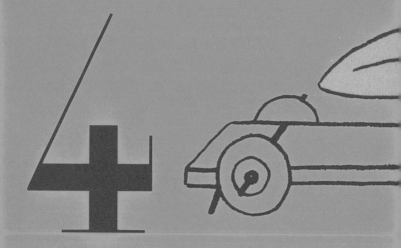

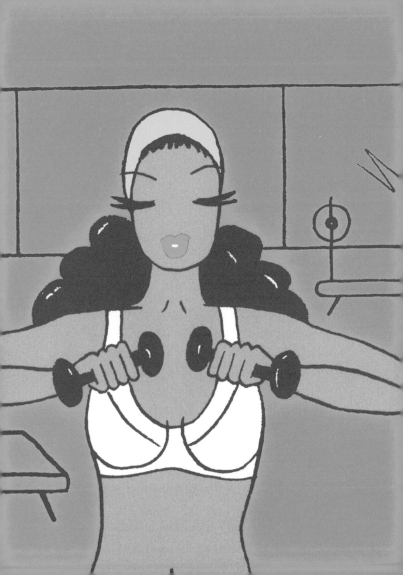

A firm and toned décolletage doesn't end with
the chest. To create a beautiful framework for your
breasts, you need to shape and define the muscles
of your shoulders and arms. Toned shoulders also
eliminate the need for shoulder pads and balance a
pear-shaped physique by adding width to the upper
body, which visually slims the hips and lower body.

Rounded shoulders are never a good look. More
importantly, rounded shoulders usually accompany a
collapsed chest, weak back, and tight neck. This all
adds up to chronic tension in the neck and shoulders,
which shows as strain in your face and keeps you
from breathing deeply and standing up straight.
Use these exercises to relieve tension, improve
posture, and reduce your risk of shoulder injuries—
especially useful when you need to push away your
many ardent admirers!

Training your shoulders and arms is rewarding. You
can get visible results in a relatively short amount of
time. Keep in mind that on many social occasions, such
as dining, people mainly view the upper part of your
body. Boost your bare-armed confidence by regularly
training your biceps and triceps. Once you strengthen

these typically weak muscles, you'll feel so proud of yourself, you'll walk right out the door and conquer the world.

The following exercises target your shoulders and arms. Practice these toning exercises two to three times a week (greater frequency yields more definition and quicker results). For most women, one to three sets, of eight to twelve repetitions to fatigue apiece, are enough to improve strength and endurance and to build those defined "celebrity arms."

A small percentage of women are able to build large muscles. If you're concerned that your shoulder or arm muscles might get too big, do just one set of fifteen to twenty repetitions to fatigue. Use a lightweight exercise band or tube that you are able to extend up to twenty times before your muscles tire. If you're happy with the amount of tone and strength that you achieve with one set, stick with it; if you find you do want more muscle, work up to two or three sets.

After strength training, stretch to ensure flexible shoulder joints. Many older adults can't raise their arms overhead. This is not an inevitable result of aging; instead, it results from not moving fully on a regular basis. But even if you've lost some flexibility, you can regain it with consistent stretching. The best time to stretch is immediately after your toning exercises, while your muscles are warm and pliable.

no. 24

"hooray for hooters" overhead press

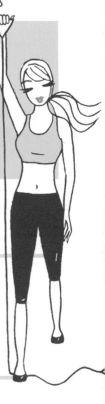

Sit in a chair or stand in a split stance, right foot forward, shoulders relaxed, and arms at your sides. Hold one end of an exercise tube or band in your right hand and stand on the tube or band with your right foot. Tighten your abdominal muscles to support your back. Maintain good posture (see exercise 11).

* Lift your right hand to shoulder height, with your elbow bent and your palm facing forward. Relax your left arm at your side.

* Exhale as you lift your right hand overhead and slightly forward as far as is comfortable, palm facing forward. Keep your shoulders relaxed, torso stable, and wrists flat. Avoid hunching your shoulders or arching your lower back.

* Inhale as you lower your arm to the starting position. (Continued)

no. 24 (CONT.)

"hooray for hooters" overhead press

* Do eight to twelve repetitions or work for up to one minute.

---

* Switch arms and repeat.

---

* After this exercise, stretch your shoulders with exercise 7, the "Queen of the World" Chest and Front-Shoulder Stretch.

secrets of style

WORK THOSE SHOULDERS! The skin of your shoulders and arms is not as delicate as the décolletage. Exfoliate regularly with a body scrub, and moisturize with a cream suited to your skin type. Remember, too, that bare shoulders send inviting messages of femininity. Strike a sexy pose by placing your hands on your hips and throwing your shoulders forward or backward.

no. 25

"going my way?" side raise

Sit or stand with your shoulders relaxed, holding
one end of an exercise band in each hand.
Hold your left hand in front of your body with
your right arm at your side, right palm facing
in and right thumb extended and facing forward.
Tighten your abdominals to support your back.
Keep good posture (see exercise 11).

* Exhale as you lift your right arm sideways to
  shoulder height. Keep your shoulders relaxed,
  your torso stable, and your wrist flat, with the
  palm facing downward. Rotate your wrist to a
  thumbs-up position. Avoid hunching
  your shoulder.

* Inhale as you lower your arm to the starting position.

* Do eight to twelve repetitions or work for up to
  one minute.

* Switch arms and repeat. (Continued)

no. 25 (cont.)

"going my way?" side raise

* After this exercise, stretch your shoulders with exercise 9, the Chest-Expanding Wall Stretch.

secrets of style

REMEMBER TO PROTECT YOUR SHOULDERS, upper back, and the back of your neck, as well as your facial and decollétage skin, from sun damage and premature aging. Wear at least SPF 15 full-spectrum sunscreen to protect against harmful UVA and UVB rays. Check out sunscreen products that you can add to your laundry, which prevent UV light from passing through the cloth and give your clothes SPF 30.

no. 26

"say no to slouch" rear shoulder toner

Stand with your feet hip-width apart in a split stance, holding the ends of an exercise tube or band in your hands. Extend your arms straight in front of you at shoulder height and parallel to the ground, with your palms facing downward. Tighten your abdominals to support your back. Keep good posture (see exercise 11).

* Exhale as you pull your right arm back and out to the side at shoulder height. Keep your shoulders relaxed, your torso stable, and your wrists flat, with the palms facing downward. Avoid hunching your shoulder.

* Inhale as you return your arm to the starting position.

* Do eight to twelve repetitions or work for up to one minute. (Continued)

no. 26 (CONT.)

"say no to slouch" rear shoulder toner

* Switch arms and repeat. For best results, do up to
  three sets of this exercise on each side, and do it
  regularly to prevent the dreaded slouch.

* After this exercise, stretch your upper back and
  shoulders with exercise 1, the "Diamonds Are a Girl's
  Best Friend" Overhead Stretch.

secrets of style

BIG-BUSTED? You probably often find that tops are cut with
lower-than-necessary armholes and big sleeves, which can
make your arms look bulky. Solve this style problem by
taking your top to a tailor. Have the armholes raised and
the bottom of the sleeves taken in to create a fitted and
slenderizing look.

no. 27

bodacious reverse biceps curl

Hold the ends of an exercise band or tube in each hand. Stand on the center of the band or tube, with your feet hip-width apart. Hold your arms straight at your sides, with your palms facing backward. Tighten your abdominal muscles to support your back and tone your core muscles. Keep good posture (see exercise 11).

* Exhale as you bend your elbows and lift both hands to shoulder height, palms facing forward. Keep your shoulders down.

* Inhale as you lower both hands to the starting position. If you feel any strain in your elbows, ease up and create less resistance by using lighter-weight tubing.

* Do eight to twelve repetitions or work for up to one minute. (Continued)

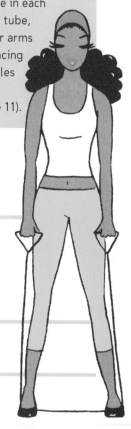

no. 27 (cont.)
bodacious reverse biceps curl

✷ After this exercise, stretch your shoulders, chest, and arms with exercise 9, the Chest-Expanding Wall Stretch.

secrets of style

A BAD FIT IS NEVER ATTRACTIVE, so a female designer has finally solved the problem of gaping button-down shirts. Now you can purchase women's shirts based on bra sizes ranging from 32A to 38D. Some manufacturers even offer odd-numbered band sizes for an individualized fit.

titbit

Size matters: A normal, healthy woman's breasts may change sizes multiple times over her lifetime. Some adolescents reach full bloom immediately; others mature slowly, like a fine wine. After pregnancy, some women's breasts enlarge; others' deflate. Some women's cup sizes vary during their monthly cycle, too. Change is normal in a woman's life, so check your bra size frequently and own a range of sizes.

no. 28

"inner goddess" concentration curl

Sit comfortably in a chair with your feet wide apart. Hold a dumbbell in your right hand. Place the back of your right upper arm against your right inner thigh for support. Straighten your right arm, with the palm of the hand holding the weight facing forward.

✳ Exhale as you bend your right elbow and lift the weight toward your shoulder. Avoid hunching your shoulders.

✳ Inhale as you lower your arm to the starting position. Do eight to twelve repetitions or work for up to one minute.

✳ Switch arms and repeat.

secrets of style

IF YOU'RE VOLUPTUOUS, try the retro '50s-style, body-hugging, or banded-waist dresses that recall Marilyn Monroe, Jane Russell, and Elizabeth Taylor. If you have a small chest or a boyish figure, empire-waist, drop-waist, and strapless goddess-style dresses are most flattering. Think of the style of fashion icons such as Audrey Hepburn and Twiggy.

no. 29

"I'm going sleeveless" triceps extension

Stand in a split stance, left foot forward, shoulders relaxed, holding one end of an exercise tube or band in each hand. Bend your left elbow and hold your left arm in front of your body's center, palm facing inward.

* Keep your right upper arm close to your torso and bend your right elbow ninety degrees. Place your right hand by your right hip, palm facing inward. Tighten your abdominal muscles to support your back. Maintain good posture (see exercise 11).

* Exhale as you straighten your right arm, keeping your upper right arm still.

* Inhale as you return your arm to the starting position.

* Do eight to twelve repetitions or work for up to one minute.

---

* Switch arms and repeat.

---

* After this exercise, stretch with exercise 8, the "Ladies Who Lift" Lat and Triceps Stretch.

secrets of style

LADIES OF THE WORLD, go sleeveless when you feel like it! Draw attention to the length and grace of your upper arms by pairing an upper-arm bracelet with a sleeveless top. Feel sexy and powerful as you channel Cleopatra.

no. 30

"top form" triceps dip

Sit on the edge of a sturdy chair that can support your weight and does not have wheels or a slippery seat that you cannot grip securely. Place your feet on the floor several inches in front of your knees. Place your hands on the edge of the seat, directly under your shoulders.

* Slide your shoulder blades down to stabilize your shoulders. Slide your hips off the front of the chair.

* Exhale as you bend your elbows until they are almost at shoulder height while lowering your hips toward the floor. Concentrate on keeping your shoulders down and stable.

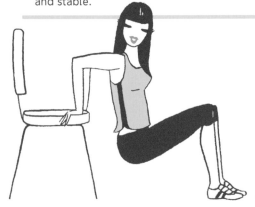

* Inhale as you hold the position.

* Exhale as you push up to the starting position.

* Do eight to twelve repetitions or work up to one minute.

secrets of style

REGULAR USE OF FIRMING SKIN CREAMS makes a visible difference in skin tone. Allow thirty days for skin to regenerate before you look for results. Scientific studies confirm that active ingredients such as copper peptides, peptide-D58, vitamin C, and idebenone all accelerate collagen production.

titbit

Female anatomy can inspire revolutions. A bare-breasted woman has long symbolized the French Republic, inspiring images such as Eugène Delacroix's painting *Liberty Leading the People*. In 1850, the French named this bosomy beauty "Marianne," and they have conventionally modeled busts of her after living French beauties such as Brigitte Bardot, Catherine Deneuve, and Laetitia Casta.

the right bra and
swimsuit top to keep
your cups from
running over

Bra-vo!

5

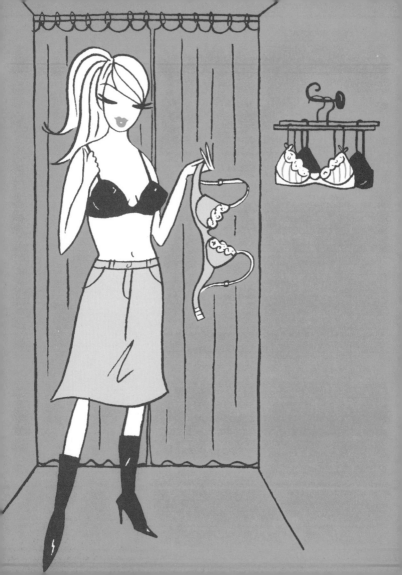

Like breasts, the bra represents many things to many people. On any given day, a bra can be a purely functional supporter or a key element in fulfilling a woman's sexual fantasies. Bras maximize, minimize, and adorn breasts in countless ways. Walking into that lingerie section triggers numerous emotions—fear, dread, anticipation, and confusion. You're excited to find that life-altering piece of sexy lingerie; you fear buying the wrong bra; you're overwhelmed by the sheer number of choices.

Seventy percent of women wear the wrong size of bra. Yet something as basic as the right bra can change your life. A properly fitting bra immediately slenderizes and improves your figure's overall appearance and keeps you comfortable. No more dragging loose straps back onto your shoulders or hiking down a back strap that rides up. For women with large breasts, the right bra can also reduce back pain. I've included info here on how to determine your perfect size and how to choose the right bra for your personal needs.

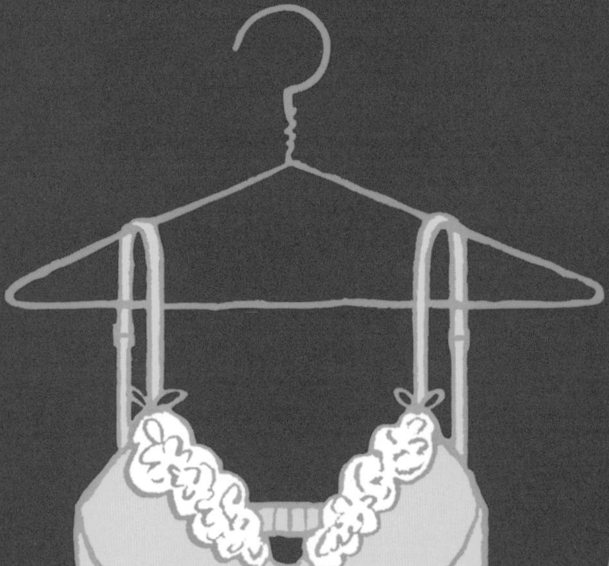

finding the perfect fit

Bra sizing doesn't have to be a mystery. It's really quite simple. Bra sizes consist of two measurements: band size and cup size.

To determine your band size, stand with good posture and place a tape measure around your torso, directly under your bust and parallel to the ground. Round the measurement to the nearest inch. If the figure is even, add four inches. If it's odd, add five inches. This is your band size. Some manufacturers are now creating band sizes in odd numbers. If you want to try one of these bras and your chest measurement is an odd number, add four inches and proceed accordingly. European bras are measured in centimeters.

To calculate your cup size, wear your best-fitting unlined or thinly lined bra. Stand with good posture. Place a tape measure around the fullest part of your breasts, without compressing your chest. Make sure the tape is parallel to the ground. Once again, round the total to the nearest inch. This is your bust size. Subtract your band size from your bust size. The difference between these two numbers determines cup size. For example, if your band size is thirty-six inches and your bust size is thirty-eight inches, you wear a size 36B. Some manufacturers are also creating half-cup sizes for a more individualized fit.

Keep in mind that cup size is *relative* to band size. In other words, cup size reflects the ratio of breast circumference to chest circumference. Therefore, the cup that fits a 32D-sized woman is not the same as the one that fits a 38D-sized woman.

Difference between Band and Bust Sizes

	cup size
* 0"–½" (1.3 cm)	AA
* ½"–1" (2.6 cm)	A
* 2" (5.1 cm)	B
* 3" (7.6 cm)	C
* 4" (10.2 cm)	D
* 5" (12.7 cm)	DD or E
* 6" (15.2 cm)	DDD or F

Throughout the world, cup sizes remain fairly consistent but band-sizing numbers vary. For example, if you're a 34C in the United States, you're a 2C in Italy and a 90C in France. International band sizes are given below (an asterisk indicates that there is no sizing standard for a size in a specific country).

United States	United Kingdom	France	Italy	Europe (elsewhere)	Australia
30	30	✻	✻	✻	✻
32	32	85	1	70 cm	10
34	34	90	2	75	12
36	36	95	3	80	14
38	38	100	4	85	16
40	40	105	5	90	18
42	42	✻	✻	✻	✻

Bra size guidelines are just that—guidelines. Just as you wear different shoe sizes depending on the manufacturer, you're likely to wear different bra sizes depending on the brand. Base your final decision on bra fit and comfort, especially in the cups.

Getting Fitted by a Department Store Pro

MANY DEPARTMENT STORES offer fittings by lingerie-wear professionals during special events and sales. Ask the lingerie department when this service is offered. The specialist measures you and helps you select the right bra for your physique. If you're looking for the right bra for a special occasion, such as a big night in an evening gown, bring your dress to your fitting. 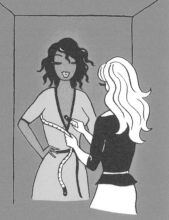 Even with a specialist, be alert to high-pressure sales tactics, particularly if the sales pro represents a particular brand. Make sure that you're satisfied and that your bra meets all the essential fit criteria described in this book.

trying on a bra

When shopping for a bra, don't be afraid to try new styles and various sizes. Experimentation will lead you to the best fit.

To try on a new bra, bend forward from the hips, put one breast into each cup, align the nipples in the center of the cups as you slide the straps over your shoulders, fasten the adjuster on the last hook, and stand up. It's best to buy bras that fit on the last hook, so as the elastic wears out, you can extend the life of your bra by fastening with the tighter hooks. Once you have the bra on, stand back and look at yourself in a three-way mirror from the front, sides, and back.

A bra that fits meets the following criteria:

✳ Your breasts should completely fill the cups: the surface where the edge of the fabric meets the chest should be smooth. If the cup puckers, it's too large. Try a demi style (with half the fabric) or a smaller cup size. If you bulge out of the cups, it's too small.

✳ The band should be halfway between your elbows and shoulders and lie parallel to the ground both in front and in back. If the band rides up your back, the band is too large or the straps are too long. If the band is slightly lower in the back, that's fine as long as it's comfortable.

✳ The center or bridge between the cups should lie flat on your breastbone. If the bridge pops up, either the cups are too small or the bra design does not fit your body. The cups may be placed too close together or too far apart to fit your breasts.

✳ Straps should rest comfortably on your shoulders. If straps fall off, try shortening them or choosing a smaller cup size. If that doesn't help, the bra's design does not fit your body. Try a T- or racer-back style instead. If straps dig into your shoulders, lengthen them or select a larger size. Underwires and properly fitted cups, *not* the straps, should provide the primary support to lift the bust.

✳ The band should rest comfortably around your torso. If flesh bulges out under the bra's band, the band is too tight and may be too narrow for your body type. Try a larger or wider band style made of a stretchy fabric such as mesh. If the band doesn't fit snugly, try a smaller size.

✳ Overall, the bra should be comfortable—no poking, pinching, or pain. If underwires jab or pinch, try a larger cup size or a different style that has a wider bridge or a protective channel or foam covering the wires. A bra that fits is comfortable. A bra that draws attention to itself while you're wearing it probably does not fit properly.

Try on a shirt over the bra to make sure you're getting a good silhouette and that your shape doesn't look lumpy, pointy, or flattened. The texture of lacy bras tends to show through lightweight fabrics, as do seams. Make sure the bra works with the sorts of clothing you'll wear it under.

titbit

In the 1950s, the enterprising creators of a new niche market invented the concept of "training" your breasts when they introduced the training bra. Fun brands like the Go-Bra, Bobbie, Adagio, and the Littlest Angel, all in sizes AA and AAA, were meant to appeal to teens. Bra manufacturers sponsored films such as *Facts About Your Figure* for viewing in home economics classes nationwide to convey the importance of wearing a bra to young female viewers.

Life is Never Simple: Adjustments for Cups That Runneth Over (or Under)

Studies show that the left breast of most women is larger than the right, although scientists haven't been able to explain this difference. If one breast is larger than the other, buy a bra with cups that fit the larger breast. If your breasts are significantly different sizes, buy a bra with removable "cookies" or pads; remove the cookie from the larger side. Try shortening the strap on the smaller breast's side so both nipples are at the same height.

If your back tends to be larger or smaller than average, buy a bra with proper cup fit and alter the band size by either shortening it or adding an extender. Premenopausal women may find their breast size changing throughout the month—for some women the change is minor, while for others it's dramatic. Buy a range of sizes for a good fit every day.

Build Your Bra Wardrobe: Understanding Bra Styles

After you have solved the mystery of which size bra you need, your next challenge is to determine which bra is appropriate for which outfit. The sheer variety of styles today can be overwhelming. In addition, bra manufacturers continue to research and develop new fabrics and constructions to improve comfort and fit. Here are some helpful descriptions:

CONTOUR AND MOLDED BRAS: A contour bra firmly holds its shape and provides symmetry and a smooth, defined silhouette without necessarily adding size. Contour bras have light padding and underwires to provide full coverage and support. They're ideal for women who have breasts of different sizes, and they are also referred to as equalizer bras. Molded bras are created by machines that mold fabric over cups to give the breast a natural look. Molded bras are usually seamless and may be either soft-cup or underwire. They are ideal for lifting and centering breasts that tend to go their own ways (e.g., north, south, or to the sides), and they work well under fitted sweaters.

CONVERTIBLE BRA: A convertible bra has straps
and hooks that let you create an assortment of
styles: conventional, halter, racer-back, one-
shoulder, off-the-shoulder, and strapless. This style
is versatile and ideal if you have a variety of clothing
styles, especially in warm-weather wear. Choose a
convertible bra with beaded or jeweled straps and
an extra pair of clear straps for the widest range
of options.

DEMI, SHELF, OR BALCONETTE BRA: A demi or shelf
bra is an underwire, contour-styled bra with the
upper portion of the bra eliminated to expose the
top of the breasts. It features wide-set straps and
is ideal for low-cut, scooped, rounded, or wide,
square necklines. This style is not recommended
if you have sloping shoulders, as the straps will
slide off. A balconette is a demi or shelf bra with
padding that enhances the cleavage. This is a great
bra for lift and separation, but I don't recommend
wearing the balconette with T-shirts. The cup lines
may be visible through the T-shirt, and your breasts
might seem to spill over the tops of the cups.

INSERTABLE PADS, CUTLETS, OR CUPS: Thank heavens for modern technology. Today's natural-looking and comfortable pads make it a cinch to enhance your bustline. If you're small-chested and want to fill out a special dress or swimsuit, you can sew in foam pads. If your breasts seem to have a mind of their own, insert silicone cutlets to restore order and alignment. If you're large-breasted and want to wear a plunging V-neck, a spaghetti-strap sundress, or a sexy strapless gown, sew cups directly into your top. Take advantage of the marvels of modern engineering to make every garment fit and to reveal your assets in their best light.

MINIMIZER BRA: A minimizer bra reduces the apparent size of large breasts (D-cup or above) while providing a smooth, natural look. The minimizer is ideal for any woman who feels that she's top-heavy and wants to balance the proportions of her physique. It offers full coverage and reduces overall size by distributing broad support while maintaining lift and separation. A good minimizer bra should not smash your chest or create a mono-boob look.

PLUNGE OR DEEP V BRA: A plunge bra enhances the appearance of cleavage because of its deep, V-style, angled cups with side padding and a thin bridge. Plunge bras are not as heavily padded as push-up bras (see below). They are ideal for low-cut necklines and a sexy, full-cleavage look. Use double-sided lingerie or toupee tape to secure your clothing when you want to show off deep cleavage. Plunge bras and other kinds of side-padded bras are also great for breasts that have lost volume and lift post-pregnancy.

PUSH-UP OR ENHANCER BRA: A push-up bra makes your breasts look bigger through additional padding at the bottom of its cups. Some of these bras, known as pocket bras, allow you to remove these pads, referred to as cookies or cutlets, if you want to enjoy your natural size. Push-up or pocket bras are ideal for smaller breasted women—especially those with broad shoulders—who want to look bustier in particular outfits or who simply want to create a more curvaceous figure.

SEAMED BRA: Any bra with seams running through its cups is a seamed bra. They provide shape and lift. The most supportive of these bras have seamed cups made in three pieces that form a T-shape, which gives more support than a single dart or a diagonal seam that starts at the bridge. The seamed bra is ideal for women who want to lift their boobs away from their waists for a slenderized contour under clothes.

SOFT-CUP BRA: A soft-cup bra has a molded cup, but no underwire or padding. This style is ideal for women who wear an A or B cup and who prefer a very comfortable, natural look.

SPORTS BRA: Your sports bra is as important as your exercises to ensure firm and lifted breasts. Minimize bouncing and preserve your natural lift and perkiness with a sturdy, supportive bra. The best designs have wide straps and broad separate-cup coverage. Studies show that bras with separate-cup coverage and straps that go directly across your shoulders, rather than diagonally across your back, provide better support. If you're very busty and one bra is insufficient to control bouncing, wear two bras at once to maximize support.

STICK-ON BRA DEVICES: Another brilliant product from today's fashion engineers, these are adhesive products that provide support, conceal nipples, and even attach entire cups to the chest without straps. They're sideless, backless, strapless, and completely invisible under clothes, so you simply have no reason for sloppy straps or sagging breasts.

T-SHIRT BRA: A T-shirt bra is made of a smooth, seamless fabric for an invisible fit under T-shirts or tight-fitting tops. It's often molded and very lightly padded to conceal nipples. It's ideal for a woman who wants a minimal look under tight tops. Larger T-shirt bras, in C cups or above, typically have underwires. Manufacturers are developing methods to fuse seams into the inside of the fabric to create a more seamless effect. The T-shirt bra, like other seamless bras, tends to flatten and spread breasts rather than lift the bustline. For more lift, choose a molded-cup bra (see "Soft-Cup Bra"), not a T-shirt bra.

Caring for Your Bras

IDEALLY, YOU SHOULD HAND-WASH your bras in cold water with lingerie soap. Regular detergents can break down elastic and lace. Avoid heat, as it destroys elastic. Do not wring or twist bras, as that can ruin the shape; simply hang them up to air-dry. If you must machine-wash your bras, fasten the straps to avoid snagging and stretching, put them in a lingerie bag, and use the gentle cycle.

Your Swimsuit Fit

Now that you've mastered finding the perfect bra, you can turn your attention to finding the perfect swimsuit. The top should not only flatter your breasts, but also provide the support you need for your activities. If you're planning to just sun yourself, go for an unstructured top. But if swimming, boating, or snorkeling is on the agenda, make sure you choose a bathing suit that allows movement and comfort. I've outlined here which sorts of suits are best for different body types. As with brassieres, though, I encourage you to try on a variety to see which styles look and feel best on your particular figure. Make the most of yourself, and dazzle them at the beach or poolside.

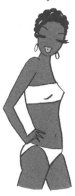

For the Small-Chested

* Bandeau tops with shirring to create more volume
* String-bikini triangle tops
* Light and bright saturated colors
* Small prints and patterns
* Push-up bralike tops with ornamentation
* Keyhole tops
* Plunging V-front or low-scoop necklines
* Tops with ruching or ruffles

For the Big-Breasted

* Bandeau tops with shelf bras and/or boning for extra support
* Underwires
* Wide or double shoulder straps
* Dark, deep colors; solids
* Lingerie-inspired designs with supportive bralike features

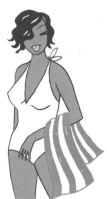

* Halter tops
* Empire waists with banding under the breasts
* Fabrics with lots of hold-everything-in stretch that aren't so tight they create bulge lines
* Side boning
* Large prints
* Athletic-styled two-pieces

For the Boyish or Narrow-Hipped

* Halter tops
* One-piece suits with cut-outs
* Angled stripes
* Ruching at the waist or through the center
* Belted one-pieces

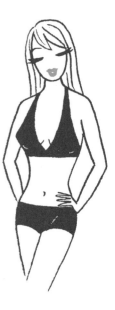

THE BOTTOM LINE: Have fun and express yourself. Choose wisely from the great diversity of today's selections. Your only rule of thumb: fit and comfort are queen. Knock 'em dead with your knockers.

Bra Longevity Tips

AT A MINIMUM, you should own three everyday bras—including at least one in nude and one in black. Three bras allow you to have one to wear, one to wash, and one to serve as an alternate. To maximize longevity, avoid wearing the same bra two days in a row. Let the elastic recover for at least twenty-four hours so it won't stretch out too quickly. Start out wearing your bra on the last hook, and then use the inner hooks as the band elastic stretches out. Replace frequently worn bras at least every six months to ensure good support. Be sure to recheck your measurements at least every two years to ensure that your size hasn't changed.

resources

Neck, Décolletage, and Bust Care Products

The following companies create exclusive beauty products specifically designed to care for the neck, décolletage, and bust at home, and they're available only through trained aestheticians at top spas worldwide. Use the contact information below to find a skin care professional near you.

 DECLÉOR
888.414.4471
www.decleor.com

 JURLIQUE
800.854.1110
www.jurlique.com

 PEVONIA
800.446.3751
www.pevonia.com

PHYTOMER
800.227.8051
www.phytomer.com

 THALGO
954.525.9665
www.thalgo.com

 TRUE
800.419.TRUE
www.truecosmetics.com

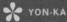 **YON-KA**
800-533-6276
www.yonka.com

Bras

Here are just a few options to help you build your bra wardrobe. The stores below represent a variety of price points, styles, and sizes, so poke around to find one nearby that fits your needs.

 AGENT PROVOCATEUR
+44 (0) 870.600.0229
www.agentprovocateur.com

 BLOOMINGDALE'S
866.593.2540
www.bloomingdales.com

 BARE NECESSITIES
877.728.9272
www.barenecessities.com

 JC PENNEY
800.322.1189
www.jcpenney.com

JUST MY SIZE
800.261.5902
www.justmysize.com

 NORDSTROM
888.282.6060
www.nordstrom.com

 SAKS FIFTH AVENUE
877.551.7257
www.saksfifthavenue.com

 VICTORIA'S SECRET
800.411.5116
www.victoriassecret.com

Sports Bras

Before starting the *Busting Out* fitness program, be sure you have a sturdy, supportive sports bra to keep your breasts firm and lifted. You'll find a great selection at the stores listed below.

LUCY (SPORTSWEAR FOR WOMEN OF ALL SIZES)

Sports bras from sizes 32 to 50, A to DDD, 52DD
877.999.5829
www.lucy.com

JUNONIA (SPORTSWEAR FOR WOMEN SIZE 14 AND UP)

Sports bras from sizes 38 to 52, B to DDD
800.JUNONIA (586.6642)
www.junonia.com

TITLE 9 SPORTS

800.342.4448
www.title9sports.com

WOMEN'S SPORTS SPECIALTIES

888.977.2255
www.womens-sports.com